SUBJECT YOUR FLESH

...and stop being a victim of your destructive desires

Beyr Reyes

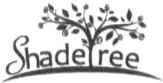

SUBJECT YOUR FLESH
and stop being a victim of your destructive desires

Beyr Reyes
Copyright @ 2013 Jennifer Minigh
Print ISBN: 978-1-937331-57-3
e-Book ISBN: 978-1-937331-58-0

Scripture was taken from the Holy Bible, King James Version, 1768 edition, which is in the public domain.

All rights reserved. This book is protected by copyright. No part of this book may be reproduced or transmitted in any form or by any means, electronic or mechanical, including photocopying, recording, or by any information storage and retrieval system, without permission in writing from the publisher.

The purpose of this book is to educate and enlighten. This book is sold with the understanding that the author and publisher are not engaged in rendering counseling, albeit it professional or lay, to the reader or anyone else. The author and publisher shall have neither liability nor responsibility to any person or entity with respect to any loss or damage caused, or alleged to have been caused, directly or indirectly, by the information contained in this book.

Subject Your Flesh by Beyr Reyes

CONTENTS

My First Experience With Subjection	**1**
There's a War Going On Inside of You	**5**
What Exactly *Is* Subjection?	**9**
In Terms of the World	9
In Terms of the Spirit	10
How To Use Subjection	**15**
Bring It Under Immediate Control	16
Exchange the Lies for Truth	17
Persist and Sustain	21
Examples of How Subjection Works	**25**
To Purge an Undefined Illness	25
To Destroy Caustic Thoughts	27
To Recalibrate the Mind and Body	29
Willpower vs. Subjection	**35**
Subjection vs. Dieting	**37**
Subjection vs. Fasting	**39**
Pitfalls of Subjection	**47**
Review Request	**51**
About the Author	**53**
Other Books By Beyr Reyes	**55**
Notes	**59**

Subject Your Flesh by Beyr Reyes

Subject Your Flesh by Beyr Reyes

Need to get control of your life?
Tired of constant dieting?
Fed up with bad habits?

Subjection is the answer that lasts.
Learn how to eradicate the problem areas in your life.
Take control of your flesh and turn your life around using the Word of God.

Subject Your Flesh by Beyr Reyes

Subject Your Flesh by Beyr Reyes

MY FIRST EXPERIENCE WITH SUBJECTION

The first time I remember using subjection, I had no idea what I was doing. Actually, it was even worse than that... I didn't see it coming and had no idea what was happening as it transpired. I found myself acting out of character doing something I had never heard of or seen before. And honestly, when it was over, I still had no clue what took place. In fact, it took several years for the realization to hit me. All I knew was that something major happened in my life, and I liked it. No... I *loved* it!

Several years ago, I spent nearly a whole week in the bed. I was sick, but yet unable to identify the illness.

Subject Your Flesh by Beyr Reyes

Every time I lifted my head or tried to sit up, I swooned with dizziness and nausea. Weak and barely able to move, I spent most of my energy crawling back and forth to the toilet. To some people, this may not seem like a big deal, maybe even like the flu, but I knew two things for sure: 1) it wasn't the flu and 2) I'm *never* sick, so this was *very* concerning.

Eventually a switch in me flipped, and with the last ounce of energy I had, I jumped out of bed and started speaking to my body like a drill sergeant. I told my body and the sickness that I was taking charge and there was nothing they could do about it. I commanded the illness to leave and my body to instantly heal itself. Whatever this was in me was there illegally, and I started cleaning house as I pulled the imaginary sickness from my belly and mind. Declaring scripture over myself and now breaking into a full sweat, I only became more determined with every breath. After about exhausting five minutes of this warfare, I collapsed onto the bed and fell asleep immediately.

When I awoke, I felt like a new person. All traces of the illness were gone, and I felt like a million dollars. This was the day I realized the extent of my control over my own body. For the first time, I put it under my complete authority and forced it to expel illness (albeit, I did so without knowing what I was doing).

So, what exactly did I do? I used subjection and the Word of God to put my body under my control. I had been learning about how there is power in the Name of Jesus and how through the Holy Spirit, we can use His authority in our lives. Also, I was hearing more about this thing called spiritual warfare. Although, I really did not know what I was doing, something inside of me grabbed hold of the knowledge I had absorbed and set me on the front line—locked, loaded, and ready for a fight. When it was all over, I realized the very basic concept of what just happened, but it was years later before I could explain that is was subjection.

This book is my best attempt at describing subjection and how you can use it to change your life too.

Subject Your Flesh by Beyr Reyes

THERE'S A WAR GOING ON INSIDE OF YOU

Everyone who has ever been alive understands the war of good versus evil. This power struggle births the finest books and movies. However, the goriest war is not on the big screen, but is within our own minds.

Paul in the Bible provides the best description of this good vs. evil battlefield in our thoughts.[1] Following is a synopsis of his depiction. How many of us can testify to this battle in our mind too?

---

[1] Romans 7: 14-24

Subject Your Flesh by Beyr Reyes

I don't understand why I do what I do. I end up NOT doing what I want to do (what is right), and instead, doing what I hate. I have the desire to do what is good, but I cannot seem to carry it out. I just keep doing the evil things instead of the good ones. When I want to do good, evil is right there with me. Even though I delight in the good ways, there is a war waging against the law of my mind, making me a prisoner of the sin at work within me. What a wretched man I am! Who will rescue me from this?

The Bible states that a mind governed by the flesh is hostile to God; it does not submit to His law.[2] Those who live according to the flesh have

---

[2] Romans 8:7

their minds set on what the flesh desires; but those who live by the Spirit have their minds set on what the Spirit desires. Furthermore, a mind governed by the flesh is dead, but one ruled by the Spirit has life and peace."[3] Jesus said, "I tell you, everyone who sins is a slave to sin.[4] But if you hold to my teaching, then you will know the truth, and the truth will set you free."[5]

People, there is an epic war at hand between our flesh and spirit. Everyone (saved or unsaved) deals with this battle.

We must pick a side in this war.

If we fail to choose the spirit side, then we run a great risk. God can give us over to a depraved mind. As a result, we would become filled with

---

[3] Romans 8:5-6
[4] John 8:34
[5] John 8:31-32

every kind of wickedness, covetousness, maliciousness, greed, and jealousness. We would be full of envy, murder, strife, deceit, and malice. People like this are gossips, slanderers, back-bitters, God-haters, disrespectful, arrogant, and boastful. They are disobedient and have no understanding, fidelity, love, or mercy.[6] Ultimately, failure to choose the spirit side leads to death.

Which will you let rule and reign in your life? Sprit or flesh? The flesh will always win the battle and rule over the spirit unless you put the flesh under subjection.

Subject Your Flesh!!

---

[6] Romans 1: 28-31

Subject Your Flesh by Beyr Reyes

WHAT EXACTLY *IS* SUBJECTION?

In Terms of the World

If you have ever watched a movie about kings and kingdoms, then you know that a king rules over his *subjects*. Herein lies the root meaning of the word *subjection*.

According to the Merriam-Webster online dictionary (www.merriam-webster.com/dictionary/subjection), following are a couple definitions of the word *subjection*:

- to bring under control or dominion

- to make (as oneself) amenable to the discipline and control of a superior

A king's subjects are those people who are *subject* to his authority. Note that the converse is not true: the king is NOT subject to the will of his people. He is sovereign and does as he decides.

In today's society, animal trainers are probably the people who best understand the use of subjection. They bring animals under their control, institute a set of behavior rules, and then continue to reign over the animal while enforcing the rules.

In Terms of the Spirit

Whereas subjection in the world deals with the relationship between two living beings, subjection in terms of the spirit deals with the conflict between our flesh and our spirit. As described in the previous chapter, our fleshly desires are at war with our spirit.

When Jesus came to earth, He was God in the flesh. God came to earth, lived, and died as a man; and therefore, He had the right to take man's place in death. Jesus was the spotless sacrifice that was good enough to cover all of humanity's sins forever. No longer did the priests have to perform a sacrifice once a year to temporarily cover the people's sins. Jesus was a one-and-done sacrifice that covered it all for eternity.

Unless you have accepted Jesus as your Savior and Redeemer, you face an inescapable and eternal death. If this is your situation, then stop right now and offer yourself to God. Pray aloud this prayer to be saved.

Dear Heavenly Father, I accept Jesus Christ as my Savior and

Subject Your Flesh by Beyr Reyes

Redeemer. I believe He died for my sins. I confess my sins and ask that they be forgiven. Please fill me with Your Holy Spirit. I declare that Jesus is Lord, and I will live my life serving Him. Amen.

Through Jesus' death and resurrection, we have been set free from the law of sin and death. Now, sin is no longer our master,[7] and we are able to live according to the Sprit and not by the flesh. We have the power, by the Holy Spirit, to put our flesh under subjection. In other words, our spirit can now rule over our flesh instead of our flesh ruling over us. We become overcomers of the world[8] and are able to put to death everything that hinders us such as

---

[7] Romans 6:14
[8] 1 John 5:4

sexual immorality, impurity, lust, and greed.[9]

The remainder of this book addresses spiritual subjection and the power we have to conquer bad habits, addictions, and evil desires.

---

[9] Colossians 3:5

Subject Your Flesh by Beyr Reyes

Subject Your Flesh by Beyr Reyes

HOW TO USE SUBJECTION

Subjection works by retraining yourself to respond differently to stimuli. It's a process of bringing your body, mind, and emotions into line with what you deem to be acceptable.

Subjection is the key to training animals, and we can apply the same principles to retraining ourselves and taming our own personal beasts.

Christians use subjection all the time without realizing it. When we get saved, we are immediately told the rules of Christianity – like how to dress and talk, where we can and cannot go, what we can and cannot eat, etc. If we stay in Church long enough, we usually succumb to the rules and change our lifestyle. This type of subjection process transpires over many years. The change is so gradual that differences can only be noted when looking back five to ten years at a time.

While the process described above works, more often than not, we cannot afford to spend a decade waiting on it—we need help now. So, where to start?

Bring It Under Immediate Control

Like with training dogs, the trainer must assume immediate control of the situation and become the dominant force. Likewise, for ourselves, the first step in subjection is taking immediate control over our flesh. This isn't the time to waiver or vacillate. The Bible tells us to not run like someone running aimlessly, to not fight like a boxer beating the air.[10]

We take control of our flesh by the authority in the Name of Jesus. The power in His Name enables us to bring our problems under control[11] and to take captive the venomous thoughts surrounding the issue.[12]

Exchange the Lies for Truth

When dealing with a dog's bad behavior, once the trainer has control and has asserted dominance, he must encourage the animal to exchange the bad behavior for a good one. Likewise, once we take captive our flesh and/or thoughts, we must replace the lies with truth. We must exchange man's ways and thoughts with those of God,

---

[10] 1 Corinthians 9:26
[11] Philippians 3:21
[12] 2 Corinthians 10:5

swap the fleshly desires for spiritual ones.

Bad behaviors arise when we live according to the flesh and begin to accept the lies of the enemy over the Word of God. The Bible says we exchange the truth about God for a lie, and end up worshipping created things (food, TV, internet, etc.) rather than the Creator Himself.[13]

Whatever issue you are facing, find a scripture that indicates God's thoughts on the matter. The Bible is the Living Word and _all_ answers are found within. Have a scripture ready for the things that challenge you most. Following are some examples.

Lie: I'm a nobody.
Truth: I am a child of the King.[14]

Lie: I can't do anything right.

---

[13] Romans 1:25
[14] Romans 8:17

Truth: I can do all things through Christ, who strengthens me.[15]

Lie: I'll never amount to anything
Truth: I am God's workmanship, created in Christ for good works.[16]

Lie: I'm a failure.
Truth: I am more than a conqueror though Christ.[17]

Lie: I can't stop eating, and I'm hungry all the time.
Truth: My hunger will no longer be for food, but will be for the Lord. Jesus said to me, "I am the bread of life. He who comes to Me shall never hunger, and he

---

[15] Philippians 4:13
[16] Ephesians 2:10
[17] Romans 8:37

who believes in Me shall never thirst."[18]

Lie: I am sick and there's no way I'll get better.
Truth: He sent His word and healed me; He delivered me from my destructions.[19] By Jesus' stripes, I am healed.[20]

Lie: I'm the blame for everything.
Truth: There is no condemnation for me because I am in Christ Jesus.[21]

Lie: I can't stop spending money.
Truth: I can keep my life free from the love of money and be content with what I have.[22]

---

[18] John 6:35
[19] Psalm 107:20
[20] Isaiah 53:5 and 1 Peter 2:24
[21] Romans 8:1
[22] Hebrews 13:5

Borrowers are servants to lenders, and I won't let spending make me a slave to anyone.[23]

Persist and Sustain

Once a dog has replaced the bad behavior with the acceptable one, the job is still not finished for the trainer. This new behavior must be continually and consistently reinforced, lest the dog fall back into unruly ways.

This is the training part of subjection. We must train our mind and body to function differently. It's about living the change, not just wanting it. Success on each day makes the next day even easier.

Even though we can take immediate control of our flesh, we still need to be able to maintain it. The Bible says

---

[23] Isaiah 24:2

that it's a learning process—that we must learn to control our own body in a way holy and honorable.[24]

If we are diligent, then knowledge will lead to self-control, which leads to perseverance, which leads to godliness.[25] You now have the knowledge about the power of subjection, once you employ it, you will have self-control, and when you persevere and continually renew your mind, you will begin to reflect the character of God instead of the carnality of the flesh.

During this training period, don't fall prey to the enemy's other tricks. Don't exchange the power of subjection for willpower. (See the *Willpower vs. Subjection* chapter for an explanation of the difference.) This slight-of-hand trick is so subtle that it's hard to see it

---

[24] 1 Thessalonians 4:4
[25] 2 Peter 1:5-7

coming. The Bible gives a strong warning: "Are you so foolish? After beginning by means of the Spirit, are you now trying to finish by means of the flesh?"[26]

Also, be careful to not conform to the evil desires you had when you lived in ignorance and didn't understand the power afforded to you.[27] Even though you put away these fleshly desires, the enemy will place them before you on occasion to see whether you are still strong enough to reject them. Because we never know how, when, or where this temptation might happen, we must stay in the Word of God and be prepared.

---

[26] Galatians 3:3
[27] 1 Peter 1:14

Subject Your Flesh by Beyr Reyes

Subject Your Flesh by Beyr Reyes

EXAMPLES OF HOW SUBJECTION WORKS

I cannot tell you what you part of your life is out of order, or how to go about addressing it. However, I can tell you how subjection changed my life. Following are instances I used subjection, sometimes even unknowingly.

To Purge an Undefined Illness

In the beginning of this book, I told a story of how I used subjection to deal with an unexplained, yet crippling illness I was experiencing. I began by telling my body and the illness that I was in charge through the power invested to me by the Name of Jesus. Having established the proper control,

Subject Your Flesh by Beyr Reyes

I declared scripture over myself and spoke things such as:

1. By the stripes of Jesus, I am healed.[28]

2. Lord, increase my faith so that I might be healed.[29]

3. Satan, the Lord rebukes you.[30]

4. My help comes from the Lord.[31]

5. My body is a temple of the Holy Spirit not illness.[32]

6. I bind this sickness and loose healing.[33]

---

[28] Isaiah 53:5
[29] Mark 10:52
[30] Zechariah 3:2
[31] Psalm 121:1
[32] 1 Corinthians 6:19
[33] Matthew 18:18

7. In the Name of Jesus, I command sickness to leave my body. I cast out the spirit of infirmity.[34]

After the exhausting ordeal and a long nap, I awoke and found myself completely healed. Since this episode, if I feel any sort of sickness coming on, I just take charge and subject the illness and fears to the Spirit. So far, it's always worked.

To Destroy Caustic Thoughts

Yes, the enemy finds his way into my mind, especially under certain circumstances. For example, after I publicly address a group of people, the devil will start whispering words laced with self-doubt and regret. He brings to my attention all the errors I made, all the hurtful things I said (never mind they were not intentional), all

---

[34] John 14:12-13

the gossip people will be burning to spread about me. Sometimes his voice is so loud and persistent that I have to start screaming "NO!!" in my head every time I hear him start to breath another slur. I refuse to let him put me under *his* subjection.

Because I now understand the enemy's modus operandi toward me, I can cut him off at the pass. When I'm scheduled to speak, I prepare my arsenal of scriptures and don't wait for the enemy to show up before I start using them. I put my fear and self-doubt under subjection right away and hold them there. If the enemy shows up I tell him (and myself) things like:

1. No weapon against me shall prosper. I condemn every tongue that rises against me.[35]

---

[35] Isaiah 54:17

Subject Your Flesh by Beyr Reyes

2. I am established in righteousness and oppression will not touch me.[36]

3. I quench every fiery dart of the enemy.[37]

4. I don't have the spirit of fear, but of power, love, and a sound mind.[38]

5. I fill my mind with whatever is true, noble, right, pure, lovely, and admirable. Everything that is excellent or praiseworthy, I will think about such things.[39]

To Recalibrate the Mind and Body

Fed up with my current health status, I was disgusted with my lack of

---

[36] Isaiah 54:14
[37] Ephesians 6:16
[38] 2 Timothy 1:17
[39] Philippians 4:8

exercise and gradual weight gain that was accelerating the speed at which my body was aging. In addition, I was battling doubt because I had expected certain things to come to pass, and yet found myself still waiting. I needed to hit a spiritual reset button—a complete recalibration of my body and mind. To physically address my declining health and mindset, I avowed to exercise every day for at least ten minutes and to eat only half of my normal portion size.

Each morning before I stepped onto the elliptical trainer, I would command my body to do it. If my body didn't feel like completing the program, I commanded it to do so anyway. (You would be surprised how effective your verbal commands are over yourself.)

My meals were yet another opportunity for me to let my body know who was in control. I prepared my plate just as before; however, before I commenced to eat, I would divide the food and only eat half. You might ask why I didn't just put half the portion on my plate to begin with. After all, you won't miss what you don't see, right? Well, that's just the point. I wanted to let my body know exactly how much I would allow it to consume. I'm in control of it; it's NOT in control of me. (The leftovers were an added benefit because they meant less time preparing additional meals.)

Every day of this subjection period, in addition to reading the Bible, I read prayers from the book *Prayers that Rout Demons* by John Eckhardt. I did this to realign my thinking with the Word of God. After quietly reflecting on the prayers, I would speak them aloud with certainty and belief. I used scriptures to drill into my head that:

Subject Your Flesh by Beyr Reyes

1. When I decree a thing, it will be established in my life.[40]

2. I am fearfully and wonderfully made.[41]

3. The promises of God are Yes and Amen through Christ.[42]

4. I bring my body into subjection.[43]

5. I put off my former conduct, the old person who was growing corrupt according to my deceitful lusts. I am renewed in the spirit of my mind.[44]

When I finished my "recalibration", I didn't have to force my body and mind to conform anymore. My eating was in control, my mind was no longer a

---

[40] Job 22:28
[41] Psalm 139:14
[42] 2 Corinthians 1:20
[43] 1 Corinthians 9:27
[44] Ephesians 4:22-23

Subject Your Flesh by Beyr Reyes

game board for the enemy, and I was a better steward of my health. *Keeping* oneself on track is so much easier than *getting* oneself on track.

Subject Your Flesh by Beyr Reyes

Subject Your Flesh by Beyr Reyes

WILLPOWER VS. SUBJECTION

Willpower is the *management* of temptation. You will yourself to not give in to the temptation—that's why it's called willpower. The temptation doesn't go away; you just find a way to deal with it.

Subjection is the *elimination* of the temptation altogether. You command your body to stop craving that food or to exercise whether it feels like it or not. In turn, the body and mind will no longer be subject to temptation, and you won't have to deal with it anymore.

Subject Your Flesh by Beyr Reyes

Subject Your Flesh by Beyr Reyes

SUBJECTION VS. DIETING

Dieting is a *temporary lifestyle change* to lose weight. You use dieting when you want to lose weight, only to gain it back at a later date.

Subjection is a *permanent mindset change*. You use subjection to eradicate the problem of overeating and gluttony in your life forever.

Subject Your Flesh by Beyr Reyes

Subject Your Flesh by Beyr Reyes

SUBJECTION VS. FASTING

Fasting is the *temporary abstaining of something.* For example, someone may fast from food, TV, or Internet.

Subjection is the *expression of control over something.*

Fasting and subjecting are powerful tools for victory. One should never replace the other, though. Each has its own place. Use fasting and prayer when you need answers, direction, confirmation, etc. Use subjection when you want to destroy strongholds in your life.

A fast is a type of sacrifice given unto the Lord, during which we make prayers, petitions, and proclamations. In other words, we choose to deny ourselves something (such as food, sweets, TV, etc.) and give it to God as an offering while we seek Him. When we deprive our body and mind of the item, it creates a longing. When we think about or crave that item, it should be a stimulus reminding us to pray and fellowship with God. This longing is a tool to remind us of how we should long for Him. The closer we draw to God, the nearer He comes to us and the louder He hears our prayers.

Don't use fasting and subjection at the same time because it will produce conflicting results. The act of fasting increases your cravings as a signal to pray. The goal of subjection is to remove the craving altogether. You don't want these two opposing things going on simultaneously.

Subject Your Flesh by Beyr Reyes

Consider the following example.

Claire has a problem with sweets and wants to give them up for good. Without the knowledge of subjection, Claire chooses to fast and pray about her situation. She stops eating sweets as part of a long-term fast. After all, she knows that by not eating the goodies, eventually she will stop craving them. She figures that she will just "fast" until the breakthrough. Claire sets out on her plan, and sure enough, after a couple months, she no longer craves the sweets, so she concludes the "fast". Not long after, though, Claire finds herself back in the same predicament, only this time it's even worse. She wonders what went wrong.

More often than not, people end up with the same results as Claire. Let's dissect Claire's approach to see what went wrong and how we can change this trap in our own lives.

First of all, Claire chose the tool of fasting, which is designed to work via her cravings. She set herself up for more work right from the start. Think about it – fasting is about prayer, and more cravings equal more prayer. She had no choice but to be faced with multiple cravings each day, when the original goal was to get rid of the cravings.

Next, Claire "fasted" until she felt that she reached a breakthrough. In other words, she let her feelings determine the course of the plan. She allowed her body to decide for her; it was in control.

Lastly, Claire stopped her efforts. This is contrary to the Word of God which says that we are to continually renew our minds.[45] If we don't, then when an impure spirit comes out of a person, and later returns to find the house (our mind) unoccupied (without God's Word), it goes and brings with it seven other spirits more wicked than itself, and they go in and live there. The final condition of that person is worse than the first.[46] This is exactly what happened to Claire. In the end, her problem was much worse than before.

Now consider what would have happened if Claire had known about subjection and used it instead of fasting.

> *Claire chose to use subjection to break the stronghold of sweets in her life. The first thing she did was tell her body that it would no longer crave them. She used*

---

[45] Romans 12:2
[46] Matthew 12:43-45

the Name of Jesus to put her fleshly cravings under subjection. Immediately she sensed the power and thought this just might work. Every time the cravings would rear their ugly head, she would cast them down and tell her body to reject them. In addition, she used scripture to fill the hole in her mind that the cravings previously filled. "Taste and see that <u>The Lord</u> is good, and blessed am I for trusting in Him."[47] Claire set out on her plan, and very soon, the cravings no longer affected her. Nevertheless, when they did surface she continued her approach. Years later, Claire is still free from the addiction to sweets. In addition, the cravings are far and few between, and

---

[47] Psalm 34:8

Subject Your Flesh by Beyr Reyes

they never hold her attention. Claire is an overcomer by the Holy Spirit. She has been set free.

Subject Your Flesh by Beyr Reyes

PITFALLS OF SUBJECTION

1. Subjecting others to our will

Once we harness the power of calling our will, mind, and body into subjection, we may be tempted to draw other people under our control. We must be careful to not fall into this trap, which leads to domination, manipulation, and abuse.

2. Not subjecting ourselves to God

We must submit all our ways to God, and He will make our paths straight.[48] When we submit ourselves to God, He will come near to us and lift us up.[49] If we don't submit to God, He will give

---

[48] Proverbs 3:6
[49] James 4:7-10

us over to our stubborn hearts to follow our own devices.[50]

4. Judging one another's subjection

Not everything is bad for everyone. People deal with different strongholds. While one person may struggle with food, another may wrestle with pornography. Therefore, the person overcoming food addictions or eating disorders may have more stringent guidelines for subjecting their flesh. The one who eats everything must not treat the one who does not with contempt, and likewise, the one who does not eat everything must not judge the one who does.[51] Furthermore, if the person who has no restrictions on their eating flaunts it in front of the person who does, he is no longer acting out of love.[52] This

---

[50] Psalm 81:11-12
[51] Romans 14:3
[52] Romans 14:15

same concept applies to all strongholds and subjections.

5. Not subjecting to authorities

The Bible clearly states that we are to submit to governing authorities, because God establishes them.[53] Furthermore, whoever rebels against the authority is rebelling against what God has instituted, and will bring judgment on themselves. It is necessary to submit to authorities, not only because of possible punishment, but also as a matter of conscience. In addition, we are to pray, intercede, and give thanks for them, that we may lead a quiet and peaceable life.[54]

6. Not protecting our new mindset

To protect our new mindset, we are to continually renew our minds[55] and

---

[53] Romans 13:1-5
[54] 1 Timothy 2:1-2
[55] Romans 12:2

put on the armor of God, so that we can take a stand against the devil's schemes.[56]

We must buckle the belt of truth around our waist, put on the breastplate of righteousness, fit our feet with the gospel, take up the shield of faith to extinguish the enemy's flaming arrows, put on the helmet of salvation, and carry the sword of the Spirit, which is the word of God.[57] We must be alert and always keep on praying.[58]

---

[56] Ephesians 6:11
[57] Ephesians 6:14-17
[58] Ephesians 6:18

Subject Your Flesh by Beyr Reyes

REVIEW REQUEST

I hope you have gained some helpful knowledge about subjection and now understand the power afforded to you by the Name of Jesus.

Now that you've read this book, if you enjoyed it, then please let other readers know. Let's share the knowledge and help people to get set free from their personal bondages.

Subject Your Flesh by Beyr Reyes

Subject Your Flesh by Beyr Reyes

ABOUT THE AUTHOR

BEYR REYES received her doctorate degree in biomedical science. She has produced over 200 publications in science, medicine, and fiction genres. In addition, she has worked in the drug industry since 2005 as a regulatory writer for major international pharmaceutical and biotech companies. (Beyr Reyes is Jennifer Minigh's pen name for the Christian genre.)

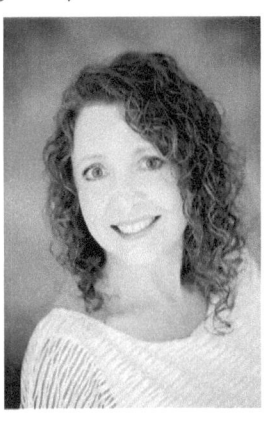

Subject Your Flesh by Beyr Reyes

Subject Your Flesh by Beyr Reyes

OTHER BOOKS BY BEYR REYES

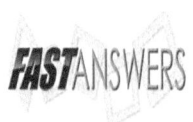

Fast Answers: Fasting Plans for Specific Prayer Needs
Want to try fasting but don't know where to start? This book had 1-, 3-, and 7-day fasts mapped out for you. Give it a try!

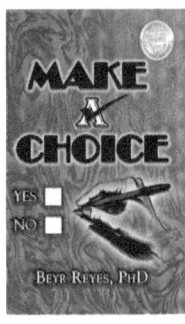

Make a Choice
What do you believe and how do you show it? This book checks your foundational beliefs and then challenges you to uphold them. Make a choice and stand for what you believe in!
Readers Favorite 2011 Silver Award

Subject Your Flesh by Beyr Reyes

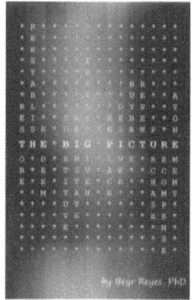

The Big Picture
For the beginner, this book is a broad perspective of the Bible that will help to place events and their purposes. For the reader who usually goes deep, this book is a refreshing step back to illuminate the big picture.
Readers Favorite 2011 Bronze Award

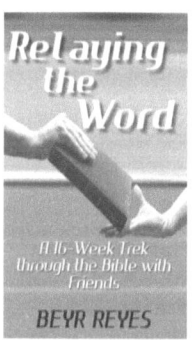

Relaying the Word: A 16-Week Trek Through the Bible With Friends
Never read the Bile? Or have read it lots of times? Either way, this small group bible study will bring fresh revelation and closer friends.

Subject Your Flesh by Beyr Reyes

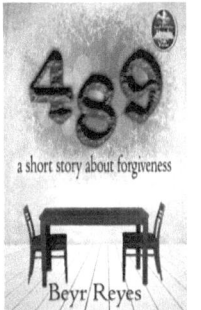

489: A Short Story About Forgiveness
If God gave you only 490 chances, what number would you be on? CSPA 2016 Fiction Book of the Year. A powerful story loaded with plot twists and emotion.

2016 CSPA Fiction Book of the Year

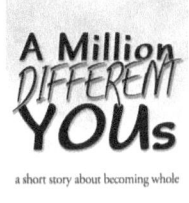
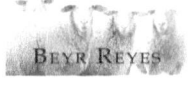

A Million Different Yous: A Short Story About Becoming Whole
Being pulled in a million different directions? Overwhelmed with all you need to be? Read this powerful story how Rachael got herself together.

Subject Your Flesh by Beyr Reyes

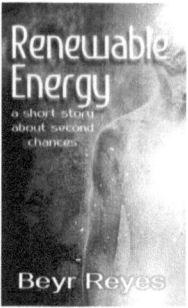

Renewable Energy: A Short Story About Second Chances
Caught in a cosmic battle for "soular" energy, will Kane find his purpose? A twist on the history of mankind through the eyes of a fallen soul.

Subject Your Flesh by Beyr Reyes

NOTES

Subject Your Flesh by Beyr Reyes

www.ingramcontent.com/pod-product-compliance
Lightning Source LLC
Chambersburg PA
CBHW030132100526
44591CB00009B/617